CW01080835

Chill Out!

How to Be Happy and Find your Calm in a Stressful World

Gemma Venn

For my Family
Missing you all.

Contents

Introduction   13

Important Note   15

What makes you anxious or stressed?   17

Plan for next time   18

Stop being busy   19

Learn to be more patient   20

You cannot control everything   21

Get outside   22

Bring the outside in   23

Get creative   24

Treat yourself EVERY day   26

A to-do list isn't just a productivity tool   27

Chill out EVERY day   28

Learn something new   29

Set the emotions free   30

De-stress your home   31

Declutter your space   32

Get on top of the cleaning   33

Organise your spaces   34

Get on top of your finances   35

Get Great Sleep   36

Enjoy a guilt-free nap   37

Hug me!   38

Get a pet (dog)   39

Make your bedroom as oasis of calm   40

Create routines   41

Switch off! 43

Brain dump! 45

Start a Journal 46

Kiss me! 48

Relax into sleep 49

Flick away the negative 50

Learn to say no 51

Break big tasks into smaller ones 52

Try yoga 53

Their stress isn't yours 54

Get that holiday feeling 55

Get it off your chest 57

Be positive 58

Affirm your greatness 59

Have a Game Plan for your Life and Success 60

Get out and meet new people 62

Eat better 63

Stay hydrated 64

Go for a walk 65

Exercise 66

Smile! 67

Create a happiness jar 68

Experiences and people, not things 69

Do what you enjoy every day 70

Be mindful 71

Slow down 73

Chew gum 75

And breathe ... 76

Try Hygge   77

Take time to meditate   78

Try complimentary therapies   80

Listen to your body   81

Laugh out loud   82

Put the kettle on   83

Stick to what's important   84

Play that funky music!   85

Go classic   86

Be grateful   87

Massage your way to happiness   88

Hypnotise yourself   89

Have sex   90

Stop comparing yourself to others   91

Visualise calm   92

Soak up some sunshine   94

Stop the Negative Self Talk   95

Try progressive muscle relaxation   96

Be generous   97

Conclusion   98

About the author   100

Also by this author   102

Special Offer   103

Introduction

It's very simple really. You are most unhappy when you are stressed or anxious. And you are happiest when you are stress-free and calm.

It's little wonder that happiness and stress are inextricably linked. Each affected drastically by the other - not just mentally and emotionally but also physically.

When you are stressed or anxious, your blood pressure and heart rate increases, and levels of the stress hormone, cortisol, increase.

When you are happy your heart rate slows and your blood pressure lowers. Serotonin, the happy hormone, is released, as well as dopamine and endorphins. These chemicals work together to relax your body, slow your heart rate and lower your blood pressure.

Although you cannot eliminate stress from your life, you can learn to minimise its symptoms - physical, mental and emotional - and you can learn how to deal with it effectively.

The biggest way you can combat stress is to make the conscious choice to be happier. Yes, happiness is a choice - most of the time. Learning to break free from the lure of negativity and to be more positive will help you to be happier, less anxious, and less stressed.

In the following pages you will find 66 tips, ✎ exercises, and techniques to help you to embrace happiness and calm in your life; to become less stressed and be less anxious.

Every thing you will learn within these pages can be implemented IMMEDIATELY. There is no excuse to be unhappy and stressed any longer.

Choose Yourself.
Choose Happy.
Choose Calm.
NOW!

** If you enjoy this book, please tell everyone else how good it is so they don't miss out by leaving a short review - a simple 5* tick will suffice.
The more reviews, the more people have the opportunity to increase happiness and calm in their own lives. Visit Amazon to review:
(UK) https://www.amazon.co.uk/dp/B07262LQJ7
(US) https://www.amazon.com/dp/B07262LQJ7
**

Important Note

If you are concerned about your stress or anxiety levels, please seek professional medical advice for long-term solutions and advanced help.

What makes you anxious or stressed?

Sit down for 10 minutes and think about the times when you felt stressed and/or anxious. What were you doing? Where were you? Who were you with?

✎ Make a list of these stressful times.

Although this can be a little challenging, maybe even a little stressful in itself, having the awareness of what makes you stressed prepares you for future occurrences.

When you know what makes you stressed or anxious, you can take steps to change your behaviour or thoughts about those situations, be prepared with knowledge of relaxation techniques for next time, or if you're lucky, find a way to avoid them altogether.

Plan for next time

Most of the time, you won't be lucky enough to be able to avoid your stress-inducing situations (and it's not the most functional approach to be honest), but you can be prepared for when they occur.

Create a calming stress-proof plan you can implement when you next feel mental overwhelm or on the brink of a panic attack.

✎ Make a list of things that help you to feel calmer when you're stressed. Quick fixes you know work for you - and if you don't have any useful ones yet, keep reading this book for lots of them.

Usually you'll have two or three that really pull you through those tough moments, such as 5 deep breaths, chewing gum, or tuning mindfully into your surroundings.

Keep this list with you so you can pull it out whenever you need a reminder.

Remember, forewarned is forearmed, so if you know you are likely to be stressed or anxious in an upcoming situation, go armed with your list of calming strategies and be ready to implement when necessary.

You may even find that being prepared beforehand actually takes some of the stress away. The unknowns don't seem so scary when you're ready for them.

Stop being busy

Being constantly busy is one of the biggest causes of stress and anxiety in our lives. However, you choose how busy you are.

Often we take on too much or say yes to things because of a sense of obligation to other people, allowing ourselves to get lost in the neverending cycle of busy. We fail to stop for a moment and ask ourselves if what we are doing is actually important - for our lives, for achieving our goals and dreams, for our happiness.

✎ List all the tasks you do and have agreed to do on a daily or weekly basis. Just looking at this list will give an indication of how busy you are, and whether you say yes to too many things.

Now go through that list a little closer. How many listed things are necessary? How many have you agreed to but wish you hadn't? How many things could you stop doing completely or delegate to someone else? - thus releasing time for the things you want to do but normally cannot find time for.

It may seem selfish at first but asking yourself if completing something benefits you, your life and your goals is key to reducing busyness, overcoming stress and anxiety, and increasing your happiness.

Remember, it's okay to say no to people and things.

Learn to be more patient

We live in a world of instant gratification, expecting everything to happen quickly, and when it doesn't it pisses us off. We have lost the ability to wait and be patient.

In order to reduce your stress and anxiety, you need to gain a better sense of time. To put this into perspective, look at the nature all around you. Nature doesn't rush. Nature takes time to produce the beautiful results of flowers, green leaves, and food.

The anticipation of a certain outcome can be exciting, and recent research has shown that using your imagination to picture that outcome can increase your ability to wait and sustain your patience for longer.

Learning to be more patient helps you to think clearer about your actions beforehand, and to ponder the outcomes possible. This calms you down and allows you to find joy in the wait.

Remember, the best outcomes take time to germinate and bloom, just like in nature, so enjoy the wait for those fantastic results you've earned.

You cannot control everything

This can be a tough one to deal with, especially if you like to be in control. However, trying to hold on to things and people you cannot change, and are beyond your control is a surefire way to increased stress and anxiety.

It is important to learn to let go - of things, people, anything you cannot change - and focus instead on the things you can. This is will result in less stress and anxiety, less weight upon your shoulders, and a calmer, clearer mind.

This quote from American poet and educator, Henry Wadsworth Longfellow, sums up letting go of things you cannot change better than anything else:

"For after all, the best thing one can do when it is raining is let it rain."

When you next feel stressed or anxious ask yourself, 'is this within my control?' If it's not, recall the above quote and let it go with a smile.

Get outside

In our busy modern lives, filled with screens and neverending notifications, we often lose touch with nature. And this could be making you sad, anxious, and stressed.

Nature is - not surprisingly - a source of great happiness, comfort, and calm. It has many benefits you can enjoy, and at little-to-no cost.

Spending as little as 10 minutes per day out in the fresh air amongst the green trees, cheery birdsong and bright flowers can improve your mood, ease muscle tension and lower your blood pressure. It also dusts the cobwebs off your mind increasing clarity of thought and releasing your creative juices.

And its beautiful to look at too!

Bring the outside in

Bring the soothing, stress-busting benefits of nature inside with some leafy green plants such as ferns, cacti, and succulents. Or add some colour with a vase or two of cut flowers.

Not only will they brighten your room (and make them instantly Instagram-able), the plants will boost the oxygen levels inside your home, thus cleaning the air to reduce headaches and tiredness.

Get creative

Have you wandered past the rows and rows of colouring books, dot-to-dots, and other stationary in shops these days aimed at adults? I'm sure you have, and there's good reason for it - colouring and other creative pursuits have been found to reduce stress-related behaviours.

Getting creative stops you mentally fixating on things, reduces your anxiety and stress, and gives you something less complicated to focus on, allowing your mind freedom to clear.

If colouring or dot-to-dot books aren't your cup of tea, why not try watercolours or oil paints, start sewing something beautiful to adorn your home, or learn how to knit a cosy winter scarf?

*** Have you wondered why the pages of this book are so plain? I have done this on purpose.*

My aim for this book was to not only teach you some great techniques for relaxation and some fantastic solutions to reduce your stress and anxiety levels, but to be a tool; to be something you can physically use to increase your happiness and feelings of calm.

If you have purchased the PDF Printable Digital version or the paperback edition of this book, I encourage you to turn these blank and colourless pages into wonderful works of art; filled with pictures, quotes, and notes that resonate with you and you find uplifting.

Yes, I could have filled this book with lots of colours, stock images, and doodles, but you might not see what I see. What makes me happy might not make you happy.

So, I encourage you to make this book your own. A truly personal copy just for you. To instantly lift your mood, make you feel calmer, and bring an instant smile to your lips.

Go on, get creative! **

Treat yourself EVERY day

Self care is vital for your wellbeing. It reduces stress and anxiety, increases confidence in yourself and your abilities, and it makes you happy and open to new possibilities.

Yet we often overlook ourselves when we are busy looking after others and running around on endless work or personal errands.

Looking after yourself is NOT a luxury. It is a necessity. You and your wellbeing will crash and burn if you do not.

Get into the habit of doing something enjoyable for yourself or giving yourself something every single day. Reward your hard work with your favourite coffee in your favourite mug, indulge in a few pieces of the finest chocolate, or take time to rest and recharge in your favourite place.

It doesn't even have to cost anything, it can be as simple as a walk in the park in the sunshine.

The important thing to remember is you can't look after others properly if you are not looking after yourself first. You cannot be the best wife/parent/employee you can be if you are not taking time to rest after a demanding day or rewarding yourself for a job well done.
You and your happiness and wellbeing MUST come first.

A to-do list isn't just a productivity tool

A to-do list can either help or hinder. You choose which.

Our busyness and high stress-levels are maintained by an endless to-do list of tasks, appointments, and notes. But a to-do list, when used appropriately, can help you to find calm and happiness by helping you to focus on what matters most.

As a general rule, a daily to-do list should fit onto a standard Post-It note, consisting of the most important 3-5 things you need to do that day. It can be less - the ultimate to-do list goal is to have a single item only - but it cannot be more than 5. For every item after that is not necessary and only seeks to increase your stress levels and move you away from happiness and the important things in your life.

** To read more about A Single Post It Not: The Key to Better Productivity, click here to go to my blog:
http://gemmavenn.com/archives/611 **

A to-do list can also boost your levels of self confidence. There is something satisfying about ticking off an item you have completed, and you feel happy at the end of the day when you look at the ticked off tasks. You did all that - what an achievement! You're awesome!

Chill out EVERY day

It has been said that silence is where happiness begins, and I'd have to agree. Especially in a world where noise bombards us on every level 24/7.

Making time to be silent and still, to fully relax and rest, every single day is not only vital for your happiness and stress levels, it is vital for your inner peace.

When you are stressed or anxious your brain is constantly bombarding you with noise - most of it completely useless and irrelevant, and some harmful such as negative self talk. This destroys all hopes you have of inner peace and a calm, focused mind.

You cannot concentrate with all that mental chatter going on, so making time to chill out for 10 or 15 minutes every day will not only help to clear the clutter mentally, it will also reduce your stress levels and encourage feelings of calm in all states - physically, mentally, and emotionally.

Practicing mindfulness, meditation or visualisation can also help you to chill out.

Learn something new

An active mind is a happy mind. Taking time to learn something new every day will not only take your mind off your stresses and worries, it will also give you a new skill to show off. A skill that brings you great joy and happiness in cultivating.

When you are fully focused and engaged in a task, as you are when you are learning something for the first time, there is a sense of calm and enjoyment that overwhelms you. Your brain is stimulated positively (this is good stress - yes it exists!), rather than negatively distracted and wallowing in anxiety.

✎ What have you always wanted to learn how to do? Make a list and then start trying out a few. Find a local class, head to the library for a Teach Yourself guide, or check out all the available resources online.

Language learning is popular and opens up many avenues to meet new people and experience new cultures. The best - and totally free - platform for this is *Duolingo*.

Or try a course in something - again, there are a lot of free ones online. Check out *FutureLearn* for a good selection of free courses covering a range of topics and subjects. Or http://www.mooc-list.com for a incredibly comprehensive list of courses across a number of platforms.

Set the emotions free

Showing emotion has long been perceived to be a show of weakness and an unacceptable behaviour to do anywhere but in the privacy of your own home.

However, this point of view is the true weakness. It takes more courage to show and be emotionally honest than it does to bury it inside you.

There is a fantastic catharsis about letting pent up emotion out - be it through crying, screaming, or slamming a few doors. Letting it out, acknowledging your emotions, not only makes you feel better inside and out, but it also reduces tension within your body and increases calm.

Emotions are better out than in. Keeping negative emotions in can do more harm than good in the long term. When you try to hold them in you are creating a volcano of emotion inside of you, which will one day, when you least want or expect it to, explode.

Long term internalisation of negative and suppressed emotions can also lead to life-changing and complex mental issues such as panic disorders and depression. For further advice on these, please consult a professional.

De-stress your home

Your home should be your oasis of calm. A place to relax, to enjoy spending time in, and to be truly comfortable.

Our need to acquire things - a visual display of wealth and status - means that our homes are increasingly becoming places of stress-inducing clutter and storage instead.

Now is the time to transform your home back into a calming living space; to create your sanctuary away from it all.

Here are just a few ways you can do this beginning today:
☺ Claim back your home from the stuff and begin to ditch the clutter.
☺ Revamp a room or two with a fresh coat of paint. Choose light colours that soothe and bright colours that invigorate.
☺ Bring nature inside with some oxygen-boosting plants and a bunch or two of vibrant flowers.
☺ Frame some of your favourite and uplifting quotes to inspire creativity, happiness, and motivation.

Declutter your space

Your home should be a place of calm for you to rest and recharge in, not somewhere overfilled with stuff that stresses you out and needs endless cleaning.

We are suffocating under all our stuff - and it's making us miserable. We are anxious about it getting broken or stolen, stressed about having to clean it and insure it, and we are so busy being busy that we don't get chance to enjoy it. Instead it just sits there, reminding us we never have any time.

A simple way to get started decluttering is to get rid of the stuff you haven't used, or even touched, in the last 6 months. Bin it, sell it or donate it. Start with a bookcase or a cupboard, and gradually work your way around the room, spiralling into other rooms until you're done with your entire house.

You are aiming for space. Space to relax and be stress-free. Clear surfaces, such as tables and worktops, make your home feel simpler, more tranquil, and ultimately, more relaxing. All of these add up to one thing - increased happiness.

TIP: Start slow - don't try to do a whole room at once. Do a shelf or two, a cupboard or a table top. Trying to do it all at once will have the opposite effect; it will just stress you out and it will never get finished.

Get on top of the cleaning

Once you have decluttered your space, it is time to get on top of the cleaning.

Breaking your home into areas and scheduling a cleaning day for each (and a day off!) you can keep on top of it all and not feel overwhelmed or stressed.

Unless you are one of those rare people who enjoys chores, creating a manageable cleaning schedule and sticking to it means you can get it all done quickly and efficiently, therefore reducing stress and allowing you more time to simply enjoy your lovely clean home.

Knowing that you can get through the day's cleaning jobs in only 10-20 minutes is highly motivating, meaning you are more likely to get it done and to keep getting it done. You've made cleaning quick, easy and stress-free.

When you skip the cleaning, allowing it to build up, and find you need to spend a few hours getting back on top of it all, you become stressed. This can be easily avoided by sticking to a simple schedule.

Get other members of your household involved too. This will make it even easier for you (eliminating cleaning-related stress), and gets it done even quicker. Now that's happiness!

Organise your spaces

A happy home is an organised home, and with less clutter, it's even easier to do. Give everything a place, and remove or rehome things that do not fit in or have a purpose.

Some say their messy desk is a sign of creativity but a chaotic workspace is distracting and a hindrance to your creativity and flow.

This can be applied to your other spaces too. You won't feel relaxed in a bedroom littered with laundry, and you won't fully enjoy that bubble bath if you're looking at a clutter of near-empty bottles and jars. And what about that bulging wardrobe, how hard is it to find something to wear every morning when you are faced with that? Declutter it for easy stress-free dressing every day!

A big organisation challenge can be paperwork. Few people find filing and shredding soothing, but like cleaning, if you keep on top of it on a daily basis it becomes manageable - and you can even learn to enjoy it!

When a bit of paperwork appears deal with it right away. File it or shred it. Don't just let it sit somewhere, gathering dust with some other papery friends. Eliminate the stress before it builds and file it away.

Get on top of your finances

For some, money and managing it successfully can be challenging. Some prefer to not think about it and keep their head in the sand rather than face reality. And others know where every penny goes.

Money and finances are regularly found to be one of the most stressful and anxiety-inducing areas of our home life. But it doesn't have to be.

Knowing what goes in and out of your bank account, and knowing where and how you spend your money, will drastically reduce stress and anxiety, which can lead to a much calmer and organised approach to money and finances.

After accounting for bills, savings, and creating a financial buffer for emergencies, you will know what money you have remaining to enjoy life with. To spend on experiences and activities - the things that truly bring happiness, joy and calm.

✎ Write down your incomes, your outgoings, and make notes of when direct debits are taken and bills are due. This will show you exactly how much money you have remaining to go out and enjoy life with.

Get Great Sleep

If you want to be happier, healthier and calmer, one of the biggest things you can do is to ensure you get Great Sleep every night.

We all need different amounts of sleep, but generally, getting 6 to 9 hours per night is what you need to be well rested, fully recharged, and ready for the next day.

Failing to get adequate sleep results in a sleep debt that will negatively affect you throughout the day - increased tiredness, increased irritability, increased anxiety, increased appetite, and a general lack of well being.

Long term sleep loss can result in some really debilitating health conditions so it is important to get enough now.

*** For some excellent tips on how to get Great Sleep and to find out more about why getting Great Sleep is so important for your health and wellbeing, get yourself a copy of my book **Great Sleep: What it is and How to get it** via Amazon:*
(US) https://www.amazon.com/Great-Sleep-Solid-Foundation-Successful-ebook/dp/B00TW8PPKG
*(UK) https://www.amazon.co.uk/Great-Sleep-Solid-Foundation-Successful-ebook/dp/B00TW8PPKG ***

Enjoy a guilt-free nap

Our busy lives don't lend themselves to getting a nap in here or there, but it is very important to find time to have one if you feel tired or unwell.

Your body always knows what it needs. It is whether you choose to listen to what it is telling you that is the determining factor.

A nap is not a luxury. It is not something to feel guilty about. It is vital for your mental and physical wellbeing.

If you are tired and stressed, listen to your body, and rest. Taking a nap has been found to reduce your cortisol levels which reduces your stress levels, which makes you calmer.

Ignoring what your body is telling you will only increase the negative symptoms you are already feeling, whereas listening to it and enjoying a restorative nap can make you feel so much better - happier, calmer, more emotionally balanced.

Hug me!

Everyone loves a hug. To be wrapped up in the warm embrace of a loved one is one of life's simple pleasures. Even a hug from a stranger can have beneficial effects.

Hugs, snuggles and cuddles have been found to reduce your blood pressure and release muscle tension. Both of these physically relax the body which reduces your stress levels, and therefore leaves you in a calmer state than before.

Get a pet (dog)

Pets are natural stress relievers, and a major factor in owning one is the happiness and joy you get from them.

Although any pet has been found to reduce stress and increase happiness, it is owning a dog that has the biggest effect on your stress levels.

Research has shown that people who own dogs are less stressed than their non-dog owning counterparts.

Additionally, if you own a dog you exercise more, you have increased exposure to nature and fresh air, and you are likely to find enjoyment in dog-oriented activities, such as training, grooming, and the social aspects of dog ownership; all of these things can increase your happiness and calm.

Make your bedroom as oasis of calm

Your bedroom should be somewhere you can escape it all and relax more than any other room in your home. It should also actively promote sleep.

Ideally, a bedroom should be for sleep and sex, but reading is also acceptable. Work, games consoles, reading other than for pleasure, and anything stimulating should be eliminated from the sanctity of the bedroom.

Banning all electronic devices from the bedroom and removing the television will not just help to promote relaxation and sleep, it will help you to build more intimacy in your relationship - if you share with a partner.

Replace the television with a digital photo frame filled with happy pictures of you and your family. Buy an alarm clock rather than using your phone, and put the games console back in the kid's playroom. Switch the iPad for a softer-screened e-reader or go old-skool with a proper book.

Fill your your bedroom with luxurious fabrics and comfortable bedding to make your bed a place you want to lounge in. Use soft lighting to soothe you into Great Sleep, and a beautifully-scented reed diffuser or candle will help chill you out.

Create routines

Routines and habits may sound dull but both have been found to not only help you to effectively manage your time and increase your productivity, but also to increase feelings of calm and to reduce stress and anxiety.

There are no surprises in routine. Everything is planned for in advance - and that's not just a time-saver.

For instance, a morning routine can help start your day in a productive yet calm manner, allowing you the freedom to enjoy some peace and indulge in some silent reflection before everyone else wakes up and the business of the day ahead begins.

A bedtime routine allows you to prepare in advance for the following day, allowing you to go to bed calm and stress-free, safe in the knowledge everything is ready to go. It also allows you time to quietly reflect on the day past, relax into sleep, and indulge in some night-time only activities.

Having routines in place and establishing habits simplify your life, reducing stress and anxiety around events and appointments, and ensure you are calm and in control.

*** Find out more about creating a successful, highly-personalised morning routine for yourself in my book, **Maximise Your Mornings: How to Create your Successful Morning Routine**. Get your copy via Amazon now*

(US) *http://www.amazon.com/Maximise-Your-Mornings-Successful-Morning-ebook/dp/B00KCSREOA*
(UK) *http://www.amazon.co.uk/Maximise-Your-Mornings-Successful-Morning-ebook/dp/B00KCSREOA* **

Switch off!

Our lives are increasingly dependant upon technology and electronic devices. It sometimes feels like there is no escape from it all because of it's constant nature, and that can be really stressful. And scarily for some, it has gone beyond mindless habit and has become a full-on unhealthy addiction to mobile phones and other devices.

Technology should enhance our lives, not bring us more stress and anxiety, and that is why reducing your exposure and taking regular time-outs from the constant bombardment of notifications and 'pings' is so important for your mental wellbeing.

Although we can feel more connected with others as a result of social media sharing, technology can make you incredibly miserable. Social media has been found to increase your feelings of jealousy, envy and loneliness, because of the biased picture it can present as reality. Increase your happiness and anxiety levels right away just by putting it on silent and out of reach, or if you are brave enough, turn it off and only give it your attention at certain times of day.

And it isn't just us that our devices are making miserable. Technology is now a commonly-cited reason for divorce and children are finding themselves competing with their parents' phones.

No longer are we giving our partners and children our full attention. We are missing out on what is in front of us, which means we are letting life pass us by while we get our fix of inane cat videos, play mindless games, and look at pictures of other people's lunch.

Life doesn't happen on a screen. Life happens in front of you. People, places, experiences. Be present and mindful of this. Give your loved ones the you they deserve, not the distracted half-listening you that tells them they're not important. Not only will this make you calmer and happier, it will also make your loved ones more secure, happier, and increase feelings of love and connection between you.

Brain dump!

Okay, maybe it's not the best turn of phrase but the corresponding action is effective.

A brain dump is a place in your journal for you to unload your brain. Every thought, plan, to-do item, and emotion; Get it all out and onto the page.

If you get it all out and face it, you can come up with strategies to tackle problems and you'll fixate less on things that have been upsetting you or stressing you out, boosting your feelings of calm as a result.

The page, like an impartial ear, is a non-judgemental place for you to release all your stresses and anxieties, enabling you to take a step back and really look at the things you have going on in your head.

If you have been avoiding something, you'll be able to think about why and create suitable strategies to move forward. Got a problem? Once it's on the page you'll be able to brainstorm solutions. Dealing with overwhelming emotion? Again, get in on the page and get to the root of the issue - or maybe just getting it down will give you the cathartic release you needed.

Start a Journal

A journal can be anything but it can also be a handy way for you to release emotions, deal with stressors and celebrate your daily wins.

Just a sentence or two per day can be enough to effectively relieve stress and and it's symptoms through the calming and contemplative nature of journalling.

✎ List 3 good things that have happened today.

Finding the good things, especially when you are having a bad day, combats the brain's tendency to focus on the negative (because it's easier to mentally process) by forcing it to focus on the positive - which in turn, increases your happiness.

✎ List 3 things you are grateful for today.

Like finding the happy things in a day, stating what you are grateful for each day helps you to appreciate what you have and those around you. This will fill your heart with joy, love, and happiness as a result.

Your journal can be anything you want it to be. It might be daily pages of stream of consciousness, it might be a continual brain dump, or it may be more planner-like. Whichever way you choose to journal is up to you but the results - less stress, more clarity, increased happiness and gratitude - are the same. So, give it a go!

** For a whole year of journalling prompts to help get you started and keep you inspired, get

*yourself a copy of my book **A Year of Self Development: 52 Journalling Prompts to (Re)Discover your True Self** via Amazon (UK) https://www.amazon.co.uk/dp/B01N9MD91A (US) https://www.amazon.com/dp/B01N9MD91A*

**

Kiss me!

Kissing not only makes you feel loved and happy, it is a great stress buster too.

Kissing releases chemicals in your body which slows the release of cortisol and other stress-related hormones in your system, leaving you calmer and happier.

Relax into sleep

If you are having trouble relaxing into sleep - because your book was more stimulating than you thought or because your mind just wont shut up - try this simple technique to clear your mind and encourage you to drift off.

Lay down, get comfy, and close your eyes. Now begin to repeat a word with little or no meaning, such as 'the' every couple of seconds. Don't say the word aloud, simply hear yourself saying it inside your head.

The meditative nature of this exercise frees you from distractions by focusing on a single point and allows relaxation to flow through you, encouraging the onset of sleep.

If you find yourself going back to the noise in your head, whisper 'not now' to those thoughts and bring your focus back to repeating 'the'.

It can take a little while at first to drift off but if you keep trying you'll find yourself drifting off to sleep quicker and quicker as your practice and confidence increases.

Flick away the negative

Not all our thoughts are useful, relevant or true, so learning to deal with them when they arise is a great skill to have to calm the mind, reduce fixation, and relieve the stress caused by negative thoughts.

An effective technique to do this is to mentally flick them away. When a negative thought arises, acknowledge it but then picture in your mind's eye scrunching it up in a ball like you might a piece of paper. Then see yourself flicking it away, maybe into a giant mental waste paper basket. You may even flick your eyes, creating an even more powerful 'real' movement to ground the visualisation in.

If the balled paper imagery doesn't work for you, try imagining the thought as a balloon being sent off into the wind on a breezy day, or imagine kicking it away like a football to a goal. Use whatever imagery resonates with you for an effective visualisation to deal with and reduce your negative thoughts.

Learn to say no

Not everything that comes your way is right for you, your life, and your goals. Learning to say no to things which are not in alignment with them is vital for your happiness and to maintain lower stress levels.

Often we say yes to things we shouldn't due to a sense of guilt or obligation, without considering the impact upon ourselves - time expended, energy expended, flexibility, and stress levels.

Learning to say no to things that do not benefit you in some way, especially to your loved ones, can be a challenge at first but in the long-term you will be happier, calmer, and stress-free.

As well as saying no, you need to learn to get comfortable with not having to explain why. Don't feel compelled to make excuses as to why you have said no. You don't need to explain yourself. A firm no should be sufficient, and if it's not, then that's their issue. Generally, you'll find those closest to you will respect your right to say no, and unlikely to demand an explanation.

Break big tasks into smaller ones

Big tasks and goals can be overwhelming and can send your stress and anxiety levels soaring. Instead of picturing this one scary big goal, think of it as a series of smaller ones - see the individual steps rather than just the whole staircase.

For instance, your big goal might be to write and publish a book. Instead of fixating on an image of a finished paperback sitting on a bookstore shelf and then becoming overwhelmed by everything you need to do to get there, break it down into small, manageable steps:
☺ Writing - each chapter, introduction, dedication, conclusion, blurb, promotional material
☺ Editing and proofreading - by chapter
☺ Formatting - for ebook, for paperback, for PDF
☺ Design - cover, promotional imagery, content images
☺ Selling - set pricing, create Amazon page, Good Reads page, Nook page, Kobo page
and so on.

Whilst keeping the end goal in sight is motivating, fixating on it and how much work it seems is not - it's stressful. Break it down into manageable steps and sections, to keep you calm about the work you need to do and to keep you working rather than giving up due to overwhelm.

Try yoga

Yoga has been around for thousands of years, and has impacted the lives of millions of people around the world. It is described as an all-encompassing practice because it can benefit almost any aspect of you - physical, mental, spiritual and emotional.

Some of the biggest benefits of a regular yoga practice include increased fitness, weight loss, an increased immune system, increased awareness of your body and your surroundings, greater inner peace, better intuition, improved relationships, and better posture.

Although yoga has it roots in wisdom traditions such as Buddhism and Hinduism, it is a non-religious practice. Anyone can benefit, regardless of religious inclination.

Incorporating a yoga practice of 10 to 30 minutes per day into your life is guaranteed to make you happier, calmer, and less stressed. It will also release any tension held within your body, boost your energy levels, relieve aches and pains - even old ones, cleanse your organs, boost your circulation, and increase your flexibility, strength, and concentration.

Their stress isn't yours

If you are surrounded by many people at work or at play, you may find that you absorb or take on their stress.

For instance, if your colleague is feeling pressured by the boss and overwhelmed by the workload, and you both work in the same department or area, you may find yourself becoming drawn in by their stress and anxiety. Remember, misery loves company! You might have been coping with the workload but because your colleague is struggling you begin to worry that you are not trying hard enough, etc. As a result, you have gone from stress-free to stressed out in less than 5 minutes.

This type of stress is not only unhelpful, it is also unnecessary. Something which doesn't affect you, has affected you. You've made yourself miserable.

When those around you are stressed or anxious or miserable, it is important to not take it upon yourself. Remind yourself that their issues are not your issues, and whilst you may feel bad for your friend/loved one/colleague, it is not your problem. You have your own and you don't need anymore!

You need to learn to deflect the stress of others to maintain your low stress levels and keep your happiness high. An easy way to do this is to ask yourself if your friend/loved one/colleague's stressful situation or stress symptoms affects you directly. If it does, work to relieve it. If it doesn't, walk away and focus on something positive.

Get that holiday feeling

Holidays. Those blissful few weeks you get once a year - twice if you're lucky.

Holidays are a break from everything mundane. They are a chance to really rest, relax and recharge. It's pure escapism from daily life.

And the holiday feeling lasts even after you return. The laidback, present feeling continues for about two weeks, infusing your daily life with a relaxed attitude, and adding the zest back into your stale relationships and dreary job.

But you don't need to jet off to Barbados for a fortnight to get that stress-free holiday feeling - but if you can then do! A weekend, and even a day away, will do if that's all you have available, as long as you go all-in on the escapism.

Ditch the phone, social media, and even the people, and get lost in reading, fresh air, and outdoor pursuits instead. Worries don't get to you when you are on holiday because you are fully present, able to relax and you can do what you want when you want - a luxury most of us don't get in our day-to-day lives. There's no stress or anxiety, only happiness and calm.

You can inject more of that holiday feeling into your life with a little preplanning. You don't need me to tell you how to book a week or two away, but are you using your days off as you could?

Every month why not have an away day, for you and a friend or partner? Pick somewhere you know and love, somewhere that fills you with joy, and then get down there and holiday it up. Eat ice cream on the pier, fight seagulls for your chips and play mini golf. Have fun, be present, and relax. You'll be blissed out for the rest of the week as a result and everyone at work will want to know your secret for making it through the busy week with a smile on your face.

Get it off your chest

When you feel stressed, anxious or miserable, an easy way to gain perspective and to increase your mental clarity is to talk to someone. Find a friend, loved one or impartial professional to verbally brain dump it all on to.

Having that sounding board available helps you to process events, situations, and emotions, as well as aiding problem-solving and understanding the why behind the stress/anxiety/unhappiness. This will reduce the stress and anxiety associated with the actions and your perceptions of them.

Just the action of telling someone else what's on your mind can reduce your stress levels - it's cathartic - and it is reassuring to know others have the same worries as yourself.

When your worries are said aloud, it can remove their power to induce stress and anxiety because you are acknowledging them and refusing to let them overwhelm you.

Remember, worries are less scary when shared, so talk it out for a happier, calmer and clearer mind.

Be positive

It's no secret that when you think happy, you are happy. In turn, if you are thinking stressed you will be stressed.

Your thoughts don't just rule your mind, they translate into your behaviour and can even be represented in your physical body.

Learning to focus on the positive is a surefire way to increase your happiness and reduce your stress levels. However, this can be challenging at first due to the brain's tendency to prefer the negative, as it is easier to process.

The more you look for the positive in every thought and situation - even in the toughest and most negatively-perceived ones - the more happiness will become your default setting, thus reducing negativity focus such as anxieties and stressors.

Instead of thinking 'I didn't get that job because I don't have the skills,' turn it on its head let the positivity shine, 'I am thankful I didn't get that job and I know the right job for me, utilising my best skills, is still out there just waiting for me to apply'. This simple reframe highlights the positivity of the situation and boosts your motivation to continue the search.

Affirm your greatness

Affirmations are simple yet powerful personalised statements that boost your confidence, increase your motivation to succeed in achieving your goals, and will increase your happiness.

There are some simple rules for writing a good affirmation that will work for you - they need to be written positively, presently, and with passion. They must also be specific to you and your life.

The easiest way to write your life-enhancing goal-oriented affirmations is to use this simple template (just fill in the gaps):

I am committed to (insert activity) (insert frequency) so that I can (insert your ideal outcome) by (insert target date).

For example, I am committed to practising yoga for 30 minutes daily so that I can lose 3 inches off my tummy by the start of my holiday on July 1st.

*** For more information on affirmations and how to write ones that will work for you, read my blog post **How to Write Bulls**t-free Affirmations** that WORK!*
http://gemmavenn.com/archives/601 **

Have a Game Plan for your Life and Success

A life without a plan leads to nothing in particular. A life with a game plan leads to achievement, happiness, and success in all areas.

So, do you have a Game Plan? And by Game Plan I mean - do you know where you are going? Do you know what you want in life? What are your goals for the month, the year, the next 10 years? What do you want to achieve now and in the long term? What makes you happy and are you doing those things every day? And so on.

If you have a Game Plan for your Life and Success, not only will you have increased happiness, you will be less stressed, more motivated, and more focused.

If you have a Game Plan you are less likely to feel lost in life, less likely to question what you have achieved over the years, and you'll be able to say no to things easier.

But what if you don't have a Game Plan? Life will be stressful, tiring, and you'll be helping someone else achieve their goals instead of achieving your own.

The good thing is that creating your Game Plan for Life and Success is simple and rewarding. It is all about getting to know you, your desires, and your images of success and achievement.

   ** *I have created the **Live the Life You Love Fast Start Workbook: Everything You Need to***

Create, Plan and Start Following your Dreams from this Moment Onwards to help you get started creating your Game Plan for Life and Success. Get started right NOW via Amazon: (UK) https://www.amazon.co.uk/Live-Life-Love-Start-Workbook-ebook/dp/B01MT82N9A (US) https://www.amazon.com/Live-Life-Love-Start-Workbook-ebook/dp/B01MT82N9A **

** For further help in creating your life's game plan, check out my blog http://www.gemmavenn.com/blog, where you will find lots of helpful personal growth articles, or consider signing up for some affordable coaching with me - I'm even giving away 1 **FREE 30-minute coaching session** as a thank you for reviewing my book.
Go to the last page of this book to find out more about this Special Offer. **

Get out and meet new people

Your social circle - or lack of one - can greatly influence your happiness and your level of success. A good social circle supports you, challenges you, and have similar views and interests to you.

If you have a close circle of friends who support you wholeheartedly, you are more likely to achieve your goals, live your dreams, be stress-free and 100% happy.

If you have few supportive friends or have a large circle of acquaintances, you are likely to achieve less, be more stressed, and be less happy.

If you need to up-level your social circle start online. Check out Facebook groups, local events and MeetUp's near you. You'll have like-minded individuals at your fingertips and with a few introductions you'll be able to build the social circle your success needs and you deserve.

Whilst meeting new people and building new relationships can be scary and stressful at first, the long-term payoffs these positive relationships have - of stress relief and reduced anxiety - are worth it.

Don't forget, the best things in life are new experiences, learning, and human interaction.

Eat better

Often when we are stressed, anxious and unhappy we crave foods high in salt, fat and convenience. We want quick junk, essentially. But these foods only make you feel worse.

When you eat well, you feel well - inside and out.

A healthy balanced diet filled with lots of fruit, veg and vitamins will reduce your stress levels, make you less anxious, and make you feel better in general. You'll have increased energy levels and be more positive, especially in terms of body confidence.

And yes, you can still have chocolate and wine. As long as it is in moderation. A guilt-free treat every now and again will motivate you to stick to a healthy diet long-term and make you happy in the knowledge you earned those treats.

Here are a few simple rules for a happier and healthier body:
☺ Ditch the junk
☺ Allow yourself a guilt-free treat or two
☺ Cut down on the booze
☺ Cut down on sugar
☺ Eat your 5 a day
☺ Gets lots of vitamins and minerals in, especially vitamin B.

Stay hydrated

Getting your daily intake of water will not only give you better skin and stave off headaches, it is vital for your happiness too.

Dehydration, even mild dehydration, has some disturbing side-effects including lower energy levels, lower mood, inability to concentrate and focus, impaired memory, increased anxiety, and increased fatigue.

Keeping hydrated will also reduce your likelihood of having a panic attack, and experiencing the symptoms associated with them.

Keep your mind fresh and clear, and the smile on your lips by getting your 2 litres of water every day.

Go for a walk

Going for a walk is a simple way to boost your happiness and increase your feelings of calm.

It is also easy to do. Everyone (if they want to that is) can find some time each day to go for a wander in the fresh air, and like a lot of the happiness boosters in this book, as little as 10 minutes is all you need to feel the benefits.

After a short walk, you'll feel mentally refreshed, have a clearer mind, feel calmer, will have enjoyed some fresh air outdoors, topped up your vitamin D reserves and will have exercised. A smile is practically guaranteed to brighten your face afterwards too.

Exercise

I've already mentioned the happiness benefits of yoga and walking, but any type of exercise is guaranteed to improve your mood and stress levels. It's all about keeping fit and healthy - physically, emotionally, and mentally.

And the good news is it doesn't have to be anything drastic. It just needs to get your heart rate up. Swimming, boxing, cycling; it can be whatever you fancy as long as you enjoy it.

Exercise of any kind will boost your energy levels, make you feel happier due to serotonin release, and leave you feeling calmer and revitalised. You are also likely to feel more confident and be left with a fulfilling sense of achievement and purpose. It can also ease the symptoms of depression and severe anxiety.

And the best bit is that 20 minutes of heart rate-boosting exercise can improve your mood for up to 12 hours afterwards, thanks to the post-exercise stress-busting endorphin surge and the euphoria it can induce.

Smile!

Largely, happiness is a choice, and when you choose to smile you are saying yes to happiness and no to stress, anxiety and misery.

The simple act of smiling can make you feel happier, even if you don't feel it at the time.

Forcing yourself to smile can actually trick the mind into believing you are happy, even when you are not - although you soon will be. Smiling is associated with happiness and positivity, so when you smile your brain tells the body to align with the smile.

Smiling releases serotonin, dopamine and endorphins; all of which make you feel good by relaxing the body, slowing the heart rate and lowering your blood pressure.

Did you know that smiles, like sneezes, are contagious? If you are surrounded by happy smiling people, you are more likely to become happier and smile more. Hows that for an instant happiness boost?

Smiling truly is a simple, yet powerful pleasure.

Create a happiness jar

When you feel sad or overwhelmed, a nice thing to have is a happiness jar. This is a special collection of memories, quotes and things that make you happy all in one place - and it is much fancier than just having a list in your journal.

✎ Make a list of all the things that make you happy. These can be things, people, places, experiences and memories. Cut up the list into strips and fold. Place these happiness tokens inside a lidded jar and put somewhere suitable in your home, such as your bedroom or desk.

The next time you feel sad, overwhelmed or just want a happiness boost, pull out a memory token. You will be reminded of one of your happy things, which will in turn trigger a whole host of other happy thoughts and memories, thus lifting your spirits and bettering your mood.

Creating a happiness jar takes 30 minutes but it provides you with months of happiness boosts when you need them most.

Experiences and people, not things

Long-term happiness is associated with experiences and people. It is memory driven - creating them and reliving them. It is not based on things.

Although you may feel happy with your new handbag/kitchen/car/phone, this initial uplift in mood plateaus rather quickly leaving you unhappier, poorer and more cluttered.

It is the people you meet and share your life with, the places you go, the experiences you have, and the memories that you create that have a lasting impact on your happiness.

Unlike things, it's not just the initial experience that brings joy, it is the memory held for a lifetime after to revisit and relive that perpetuates that happiness.

Going forward, for a happier and a more meaningful life, make your choices about experiences and release yourself from the pull of the short-term fix an object provides. You'll also be more mindful of your choices, build better relationships with people, and set a better example for your children.

Do what you enjoy every day

✎ What makes you feel calm when you're stressed? What makes you feel relaxed when you're overwhelmed? What makes you happy? What do you enjoy doing? What hobbies do you have and what things would you like to try? Make a list of these things.

We often get lost in the busyness and demands of our daily life that we fail to stop and ask ourselves if what we are doing is making us happy, or contributing positively to our wellbeing and inner peace. Most of the time, sadly the answer is no - but you can change that.

You may have heard the phrase 'do what you love'. Well, it has meaning beyond just your career and working life. It extends to your free time too.

✎ Look at the list you have made, and ask yourself how many of these happy and joyful things you are doing every day. If you are not spending at least an hour a day doing something (or some things) you love then you are not spending your time wisely. You are missing out on opportunities not just to be happy, you are missing out on the enjoyment of life.

Going forward, start to make your days more about these things. Do more of them and for good periods of time. Try new things that interest you too.

Remember, you only get one life so make sure you enjoy it.

Be mindful

Mindfulness has become increasingly popular in recent years, and it is easy to see why when you consider the benefits of a mindfulness practice.

Mindfulness improves your wellbeing, improves your mental health, and improves your physical health. Along with meditation, it has been described as the yoga of the mind for its all-encompassing benefits.

Mindfulness can increase life satisfaction, helps you to find joy in the smallest pleasures, increases pleasure in all tasks, decreases anxiety and reduces stress, changes your perspective towards others and yourself, increases self awareness, reduces negative mental fixation, lowers your blood pressure and relieves chronic pain, and improves sleep. It can also stave off the development and help in the treatment of disorders such as depression, panic, substance abuse, and eating disorders. It really does have benefits for all!

The best part is that mindfulness isn't complicated and anyone can learn the skills needed to become more mindful. It is all about tuning in to the little things and being completely present during the task at hand and throughout the day.

** Look out for my upcoming book **Mindfulness: An Introduction to for Personal Success and Wellbeing**.
Subscribe to my Amazon or Good Reads pages to be notified when it's available to pre-order:

Amazon (US) https://www.amazon.com/-/e/ B01LXL25SC
Amazon (UK) https://www.amazon.co.uk/-/e/ B01LXL25SC
*Good Reads https://www.goodreads.com/author/ show/11356574.Gemma_Venn ***

Slow down

In this modern world, we are are constantly busy and always on the go. We rush from place to place, never finding time to slow down, let alone stop.

But you need to take the pressure off; you need to slow down otherwise you will never be able to find the calm and inner peace you so desperately need for a happy life.

Make a conscious effort to slow down, to notice the things you usually rush past, and learn enjoy the calming effects of less busyness.

Mindfulness and meditation can help you to slow down too.

When you next feel like you are rushing about and have have been on the go all day, take 5 minutes to slow down with this simple exercise.

Tune into yourself and pick one action or feeling. Focus and be aware of the feeling of your chest moving up and down with your breath, how your feet feel as you walk along, or how fresh the recently cut grass smells. What do you notice? What memories or experiences or thoughts are triggered as you focus on this one thing? Savour the joy you feel, the calmness that soothes your busy mind, and the strength of your senses as a result.

When you slow down, you are allowing your mind to be fully present in the moment, and to be fully aware of yourself and your surroundings, which releases tension in your body and frees your mind.

Chew gum

Chewing gum has been a dietician's secret for years for helping to trick your body into believing it has been fed, but it can also affect your stress levels.

It has been found that when you chew gum, the cortisol levels in your body are reduced which in turn reduces your stress levels.

Reduced stress levels for less than £1?! Well, there's a bargain!

And breathe ...

How many times have you been told to 'just breathe!' when you are stressed out, angry or irritable? Lots, no doubt. Well, there is good reason for it.

Breathing on purpose and consciously taking deeper breaths reduces your cortisol levels which reduces your anxiety and stress levels.

A few deep breaths in a moment of high stress, high anxiety, or elevated anger can help to soothe your nerves and clear your mind enough to help you to see through the cloudiness and make a better decision. Deep breathing also slows your heart rate and lowers your blood pressure, countering the stress effects.

Take 5 minutes now to focus on your breath - and use this exercise when you need to calm down.

Focus on your breath. Feel it coming into your body through your nose, inflating your chest, pulling in your belly and flowing to your extremities. Feel the opposite effect and the flood of calm as you breathe out through your mouth. Repeat until you feel relieved of your anxieties, calmer than the Dalai Lama and as light as a feather that might drift off on the breeze.

Try Hygge

Hygge has been increasingly popular over the last year and it's easy to see why - it is all about happiness and enjoying life; its about being present and appreciating the small pleasures.

Hygge is a Danish concept all about creating a cosy, comfortable space to relax through the cold winter. Think warm blankets, chunky jumpers, open fires, warm bowls of soup, and reading by a rainy window. It's new pyjamas, candlelight, red wine, cuddles and casseroles.

But the concept can be adapted to any season - not just the long and frozen Danish winters - bringing happiness and joy throughout the year.

In summer, think barbecues with family, paddling in the sea, the smell of the earth after a summer shower, and building sandcastles with the kids.

In Autumn, think the crunch of fallen leaves, the changing rainbow of colours in the trees, cups of hot chocolate with melting marshmallows, and roasting chestnuts.

In spring, think vases of daffodils and tulips, the refreshing clear air after a rain shower, the lush green of the trees, and the cuteness of newly born lambs.

Hygge is not just a concept, it can be a way of life too; Focus on the present, enjoy life and all the small pleasures it brings, and relax in a comfortable space with loved ones.

Take time to meditate

Meditation has been described as mental yoga, with benefits far exceeding most other relaxation techniques.

There are many different types of meditation, each teaching a different way to practise. But whichever way you choose to meditate, whichever way works for you, will give you the same stress-relieving and calming benefits.

A few minutes of meditation each day is all you need to reduce your stress levels and ease your anxiety, and long-term daily practice has been found to make you more resilient to stress as it positively alters the brain's neural pathways.

Meditation is really simple and anyone of any age can be taught to meditate successfully, even children.

This basic practice will give you the perfect introduction.

Sit comfortably on a firm chair with your feet on the floor, your back straight, and your eyes closed. Focus on the your breath - the flow as it comes in and goes out, like the waves at the beach. Be silent, be still. Allow thoughts to come and go - acknowledge them but do not fixate on them - like fluffy clouds floating on a summer breeze. Stay like this for as long as you like.

After a suitable time for you has passed, begin to rouse your body and mind from your relaxed state. Start to notice your limbs, your surroundings, and your thoughts once again. Finally open your eyes and enjoy your calmer, clearer and happier state that you have created with your meditation practice. Repeat daily to maintain reduced stress levels and increased calm.

Try complimentary therapies

Complimentary therapies, including aromatherapy, reflexology, reiki, acupuncture and cupping, all have stress-reducing and happiness boosting benefits for those who practise them.

Complimentary therapies have had a bit of a bad press over the years, and have acquired a new age hippy-dippy image that can turn some people away from trying them out. However trying a few out may be beneficial to you. Yes, there are bound to be some that may not suit you, but you may be even more surprised to find some that do. Read about and try a few that resonate with you, and make time to practise the ones you find work.

All of the complimentary therapies have their own specific benefits, in addition to all of them being able to help you to remain calm and stress-free in your daily life.

For instance, aromatherapy has something for everyone and can be as simple as purchasing a few essential oils to dot on your pulse points or simply inhale. A good one to have to hand is lavender, which has been consistently shown to lower stress levels.

Listen to your body

Your body always knows what is needs. It is always giving you feedback. Whether you listen to what it's telling you is another thing.

Stress and anxiety have effects not just on your mind and emotions, they have physical symptoms too. Taking time to tune into your body and seek out these symptoms can tell you how much or how little the stress and anxieties of life are affecting you.

Mentally you may not feel too stressed, but your body may tell a different story. Work from your toes upward and notice where you feel tightness, achiness, and looseness. Pay close attention to your neck, shoulders and spine as these are the areas stress and tension can be felt most.

Once you know where and how the stress is affecting your physical body, you'll be able to take steps to release it through massage, deep breathing, and yoga.

Laugh out loud

We write LOL a lot but how many times a day do you actually do it? Hardly any.

Children laugh heartily, even at the more mundane and small things, yet as adults we have lost this ability to laugh with our entire being. We have become too serious and it is not doing us any favours.

A good belly laugh doesn't just lighten and brighten your face, it eases the mental load. When you laugh, your cortisol levels are reduced and hormones called endorphins surge through your system, thus reducing your stress levels and positively boosting your mood.

Laughter can also reduce the physical symptoms of stress such as fatigue.

Laughter has other positive effects too, such as helping you to build better and stronger relationships with existing friends, as well as helping with forming new ones. This is because your laughter makes you more appealing, as you are perceived as being more positive and the type of person people want to know and love.

So, do as children do and laugh freely and as often as possible. Watch your favourite comedians, comedy shows and funny films, read something humorous, and meet up with friends for an afternoon of happiness.

Put the kettle on

Putting your feet up with a cuppa feels good because it is good!

Drinking tea is a centuries old cure for a lot of things and modern science can now tell us why.

Black tea is an antioxidant, which apart from tasting great, relieves stress by reducing cortisol levels and promoting feelings of relaxation.

And it's not just stress that tea can help alleviate, it works on anxiety and nerves too. Tea has been found to increase the number of neurotransmitters in the brain which help to balance your mood.

Tea has also been scientifically found to have similar effects to meditation by stimulating alpha waves in your brain. Alpha waves are associated with deep relaxation and are present during deep relaxation and meditation states.

So, go on, put the kettle on and make yourself a nice cuppaT.

Stick to what's important

I want to share with you one of the most game-changing statements I have ever heard, and it's something we all need to listen to, and bear in mind in this busy world. Are you ready? Here it is:

> You can do ANYTHING but you can't do EVERYTHING.

Take a few moments and let that sink in. Read it a few more times, say it aloud.

> You can do ANYTHING but you can't do EVERYTHING.

Our lives are filled with things to do, people to see, places to go, and stuff to buy, but how much of that busyness is truly important?

Happiness, reduced stress and inner peace comes when you focus on what is important to you, your values and your life. Your important things are the 'anything'. These are the things you should be focusing on every day, before everything else.

✎ What are the most important things in your life? Family, friends, keeping fit, painting, maintaining passionate relationships? Write them down, maybe add a few specifics or some reasons why. When you know what they are, it's easy to focus on them every day.

Play that funky music!

Music can be an incredibly uplifting medium, capable of not only boosting your mood and energy levels but it can also trigger some of your happiest memories.

Music is so personal. It can produce so many different feelings and responses in each listener, including happiness and calm.

No matter what your mood, there's always something appropriate to accompany it or something to turn it on its head, such as music to soothe, music for love, music for sadness, uplifting music, music to get you up and on your feet.

Music doesn't just have emotional and mental benefits, it has physical benefits too. Listening to soothing music can lower your blood pressure, lower your heart rate and reduce your feelings of anxiety. Music also releases stress and its symptoms by triggering the body's biochemical stress reducers.

It's not just conventional music that works. Nature sounds such as bird and whale song have the same beneficial effects.

✎ What songs make you feel good? What songs make you feel happy, make you want to dance, and fill you with joy? Create a playlist or two for when you next feel sad, anxious or stressed.

Go classic

Classical music has been found to have many benefits, including reducing your stress levels, boosting your memory, and helping to fight the symptoms of depression.

Classical music has also been found to reduce pain, spark creativity and boost your ability to learn.

Listening to classical music before bed will also send you off to sleep by lowering your body temperature, reducing your blood pressure, slowing your heart rate and calming your breathing.

With all those benefits, it makes sense to switch radio stations!

Be grateful

Keeping a gratitude journal is a great way to remind you of all the good things in your life. These can be people, places, experiences, anything that has ever sparked joy within you or regularly makes you feel happy and thankful.

And don't forget that it's not always the big things that bring the most happiness and joy. The littlest things can sometimes bring the biggest smiles, such as your baby's contented milky face as they sleep, the tired smile on your son's face after his first day at school, the smell of freshly cut grass, or the perfect taste of the first freshly-picked home-grown strawberry.

A gratitude journal is also a good place for you to celebrate your accomplishments, such as passing an exam, learning a new skill, or finally mastering something you have found challenging in the past.

Being grateful keeps your brain focusing on the positive and helps you to move past any feelings of negativity or stress.

When you next feel stressed, pull out your gratitude journal and remind yourself of what really matters. Most of the time, the things you worry about daily aren't important in the long run.

Massage your way to happiness

Have a massage. Well, doesn't that just sound like the most luxurious way to reduce your stress levels? It is, and it definitely will!

You don't need to find yourself oiled up underneath the firm hands of a massage therapist - although by all means do, you deserve it! - to reap the benefits of massage.

Self massage can be an effective way to relieve stress and increase your feelings of calm and tranquility too. Check out Youtube for some excellent how to videos to get you started.

Massage alleviates aches and pains, and removes tension held within the body, which is often the physical representation of mental stress and anxiety. These stress symptoms are felt most in the neck, shoulders and spine.

A massage feels good (no matter who des it), relaxes you and eradicates physical symptoms of stress, but it also improves body confidence and betters your body image. And what woman doesn't want a little body confidence boost now and again?!

Hypnotise yourself

We can't all call upon the services of Paul McKenna to help reduce our stress and anxiety, but you can learn self hypnosis to help with these things - as well as a whole host of others.

Self hypnosis has been scientifically proven to calm your nerves, reduce stress and reduce state anxiety, such as the fears held around giving birth or having surgery.

It can also help you to overcome any limiting beliefs you have that are hindering your success, and it teaches you the vital skill of 'switching off' in a constantly busy world.

And the happiness-boosting benefits don't just end there. Self hypnosis can help you to sleep better, increase your self esteem, let go of painful or harmful memories, strengthen your mental state, help with addictions such as smoking, can minimise hot flushes, and help you to deal with physical and emotional pain.

Check out Youtube for some how to and introductory self hypnosis videos.

Have sex

Not only is sex great for increasing body confidence, and increasing intimacy and strengthening bonds in relationships, it is a stress-reliever guaranteed to put the smile back on your face.

Having sex has been scientifically shown to decrease your blood pressure, relieve tension, alleviate the symptoms of colds and flu, and reduce stress.

Sounds like a few good reasons to have an early night, right?

Stop comparing yourself to others

An instant way to increase happiness, reduce your stress levels and boost your confidence is to stop seeing everyone around you as competition and stop the constant comparison.

Comparing yourself to others, who lead completely different lives with a completely different set of determining factors, is a recipe disaster. You wouldn't compare an apple to an orange, so why compare yourself with another person?

You are original; unique. There is only one you. No one else can be you or live your life or make the same decisions. Embrace this and you'll live a happier life.

Visualise calm

A calm mind equals a calm body, and vice versa. But in the busy 24/7 world we live in, a calm anything can sometimes seem challenging and far away.

A simple practice to clear your mind and promote happiness and calm, is to use visualisation. This is you mentally focusing on something to bring about serenity and inner peace.

Imagining the waves crashing on the shoreline and then retreating, taking with it the debris, is a really simple and effective method of visualisation. Let me take you through it.

Sit comfortably or lie still. Conjure up a vivid image of the ocean waves coming in and going out from the shore in your mind's eye. Focus on nothing but creating this image. Hear the sounds of the waves crashing on the sand, and the rushing retreat of the water and the small stones it takes with it. Feel the cool ocean mist upon your face and taste the saltiness of it on your lips. Really invest yourself in this imagery. Make it as vivid as possible.

Once you have the image clear and focused in your mind, match the waves to your breath. On the inhale feel the water rushing inwards, flooding your body and mind with freshness. On the exhale feel the water retreating, taking with it any negativity, stress and sadness you have been holding onto.

Repeat this image-to-breath combination for as long as you wish to, rousing yourself slowly when you feel completely calm and ready to rejoin the day with a clear mind and renewed vigour.

If you prefer, there are many guided visualisations you can try online. *Ask Google or search Youtube for one that suits you.*

Soak up some sunshine

Give yourself an instant boost of happiness with some time in the sun.

As little as 15 minutes per day, will send your vitamin D levels soaring - enough to stave off the increasing cases of rickets - and it will also increase your serotonin levels (that's the happiness hormone) thus reducing seasonal sadness, and it's more intense older brother, Seasonal Affective Disorder.

Catching some rays (safely, under a layer of good SPF) will also reduce tiredness by decreasing melatonin levels (that's the sleep hormone affected by light).

You can also bring the sunshine inside with a real light lamp for an extra boost of happiness; Perfect for when it's raining outside.

Stop the Negative Self Talk

Self talk is the conversation with ourselves that is always going on inside your head. This can be positive or negative, and can greatly affect your confidence and how you see yourself.

A lot of this chatter can be negative and filled with untruths, so it is important to recognise this for a happier life.

Whenever you find yourself picking on yourself or criticising yourself, take a step back from those useless thoughts and reframe them in a more positive light.

For instance, you might find yourself peering in the mirror and critiquing your appearance. Instead of picking out the spots or the dark circles, focus instead on the beautiful smile and the sparkly eyes.

The more you do this, the easier it will be to think more positively on a regular basis, thus increasing happiness, your feelings of self worth, and your confidence.

Try progressive muscle relaxation

Progressive muscle relaxation is exactly what it says it is - it's the process of easing tension from your tight muscles, gradually.

Starting at your feet and working your way up, or starting at your head and working your way down, gradually relaxing the muscles as you go is a simple way to relieve the physical symptoms of stress and anxiety.

The calmness of a peaceful body as a result of progressive muscle relaxation allows your mind to Chill Out as a result; removing stressful thoughts, negative fixations and promoting inner peace and the ability to think clearly.

You can practice this simply yourself or you can use a guided relaxation practice. *Youtube has a few good ones to try for free, if you wish to try progressive muscle relaxation.*

Be generous

The act of giving something - be it a donation to charity, some time for volunteering, or a gift to a loved one - has been found to not only increase your happiness, but the happiness of those you are bestowing your gift upon.

Focusing on others and taking action to aid them in some way takes your mind off your own problems (and minimises them in most cases) and fills you with a sense of accomplishment, which leaves you feeling rewarded and more likely to repeat the generous act.

Being generous has also been found to create better and stronger relationships, and has even been related to living longer.

Conclusion

As you have found in this book, there are many ways (well, 69 to be precise), most of them very simple and free, to reduce your stress and anxiety levels, increase your happiness and leave you feeling calm in this busy world.

I have shared my knowledge with you, but the only way you will increase the happiness and calm in your life is to take action on your new knowledge.

Change only happens when you make it happen, right? So, get out there and act on what you now know.

The only thing standing in the way of your happiness and calm is you. So, don't be an obstacle, get out of your way and help yourself to become the Best You Can Be today!

** If you enjoyed this book, please tell everyone else how good it is so they don't miss out, by leaving a short review - a simple 5 star check will suffice!
The more reviews my book gets, the more people will have the opportunity to increase happiness and calm in their own lives.
Visit Amazon to review this book NOW:
(UK) https://www.amazon.co.uk/dp/B07262LQJ7
(US) https://www.amazon.com/dp/B07262LQJ7
**

** Share your journey to happiness and calm with other like-minded individuals and with myself on

my Facebook page: <u>http://www.facebook.com/</u>
<u>personaldevelopmentwithgemma</u> **

About the author

Hey, I'm Gemma and I have two passions in life - words and personal development. I have been lucky enough to have been able to create a career combining the two.

I have written a number of personal development books and I am always working on my next one! You can follow me on my Amazon pages, as well as on Good Reads:
Amazon (US) https://www.amazon.com/-/e/B01LXL25SC
Amazon (UK) https://www.amazon.co.uk/-/e/B01LXL25SC
Good Reads https://www.goodreads.com/author/show/11356574.Gemma_Venn

You can regularly see my work on the popular LifeGrid Magazine too, http://www.lifegrid.com.au/profile/gemma+venn/

I am also an experienced personal development coach. I offer affordable one-to-one sessions to those wishing to have a helping hand with the creation and actioning of their Game Plan for Life and Success. It is for those serious about making positive changes to Live a Life they Love. If this sounds like you, contact me now via my coaching page http://www.gemmavenn.com/coaching

I am also a wife, a mother of 2 kids under 5, a psychology graduate, an avid reader, a BuJo minimalist, a lover of cake, and a Scotland explorer. I am currently learning Danish, I enjoy reading and writing daily and I am trying to reinforce the daily habit of meditation and yoga.

To find out more about me and the services I offer, visit my website http://www.gemmavenn.com and my Official Facebook page: http://www.facebook.com/personaldevelopmentwithgemma

You can also follow me on:
☺ Instagram http://www.instagram.com/glvenn
☺ Twitter http://www.twitter.com/litchickuk

** I am available as a speaker for hire. Online and in-person. All opportunities considered. If you like how I write, you'll like how I speak. Having had speaker training from some inspirational TED speakers, I have the ability to inspire, motivate, and make people laugh whilst sharing personal experiences and sharing my wisdom. If you are interested in hearing me speak or booking me for your upcoming event, please email me directly at glvenn@yahoo.com ***

** If you have a blog, you are writing a book, have a podcast or something similar and you are looking for a little contribution magic, I am always happy to do guest posts and interviews, and will consider all writing opportunities, joint and stand-alone. Email me direct to discuss anything further glvenn@yahoo.com ***

Also by this author

☺ A Year of Self Development: 52 Journal Prompts to (Re)Discover You
☺ Live the Life You Love: The Fast Start WorkBook
☺ Great Sleep: What it is and How to get it
☺ Maximise your Mornings: How to Create a Successful Morning Routine
☺ Shared Wisdom: Tips for your Personal Development Journey
☺ Be All you Can Be: The Best of Peak Pathways

All these titles are available on Amazon
http://www.amazon.com/author/gemmavenn

Special Offer

I am an experienced Personal Development Coach and I help people just like you to create their Game Plan for Life and Success every single day - and in an affordable way.

I'm giving away 1 **FREE 30-minute coaching session** to discuss improving happiness and calm in your life, to EVERY READER who leaves a review for this book on Amazon as a thank you.

It's the perfect risk-free way for you to try coaching with me.

To redeem this offer and to book your free session, simply email me using the link on my coaching page: http://www.gemmavenn.com/ coaching.
DON'T FORGET to quote the code KEEPCALMOFFER and include a copy of your review submission page to verify your review.

To find out more about coaching opportunities available with me, visit my website http:// www.gemmavenn.com/coaching

http://www.GemmaVenn.com

34341082R00061

Printed in Great Britain
by Amazon